MW01295028

THE MEMORY CURE: MEMORY LOSS PREVENTION AND EFFECTIVE BRAIN CURE FOR RAPID RECOVERY

50 Neurobic Exercises To Improve Short Term Memory, Boost, Train Your Brain And Increase Mental Fitness

AUSTIN COFFEY

Copyright © 2019 Austin Coffey

All rights reserved.

ISBN: 9781093213072

Table of Contents

Description:

Many of us don't take the signs of memory loss for granted and regret when the consequences come. The common signs of the issue can be something to laugh at. But forgetfulness can develop into dementia, long-term memory loss, or even Alzheimer's. Have you been struggling with memory loss? Want to know how to cope with memory loss?

Within this book, you will be able to gain access to memory loss cure methods and neurobic exercises to help you prevent memory loss and improve memory. What's more, this book **contains secrets that have never been released** about the memory cure.

WHY WILL YOU BUY THIS BOOK INSTEAD OF ANOTHER?

- **Secret tips** for successful memory loss prevention and treatment such as: Step by step ways to prevent and cure memory loss with medication, diet and lifestyle.
- **Coping strategies for memory loss to practice daily** and benefits of meditation with memory enhancement. Mistakes that will sabotage your memory.
- **How to care for someone** with memory impairments for family and caregiver.

- All neurobic exercises gives the reader the methods they need to improve their memory. In some cases, the memory loss cannot be helped because it may be hereditary, but **it can be slowed down with the practice of these exercises**.
- You can find out information about neurobic exercises with understandable guides. **You can't find duplicate exercises**.
- And of course, much, much more!

Those who needs this book:

- Those who have trouble remembering the little things and are starting to forget things and have short term memory loss issues that they can't explain.
- Those who got diagnosed for any of memory impairment.
- Those who have a serious problem due to some medical illness known as dementia and Alzheimer.
- Those who want to find ways to help improve their memory and brain retention and concentration.
- Families with relatives suffering any symptom of dementia who are seeking help.
- Members of medical organizations who need to generalize knowledge about memory loss, its consequences and how to deal with it in an early timeframe.

This book provides information on the following:

- Fundamentals of memory loss and all of its related impairments

- How dementia relates to Alzheimer's

- How to cure and prevent memory loss effectively

- How to help people with memory impairments

- 50 neurobic exercises brain cure - simple, unique brain exercises for adults that can be done anywhere, anytime and then used to help you to train and boost your brain, improve short term memory, neural functions and broaden your memory

CHAPTER I: INTRODUCTION

Our brain records stories and experiences to store the moments of our life. That includes how we feel, as well as the things we touch, smell, and taste. It is a part of life no one wants to mislay.

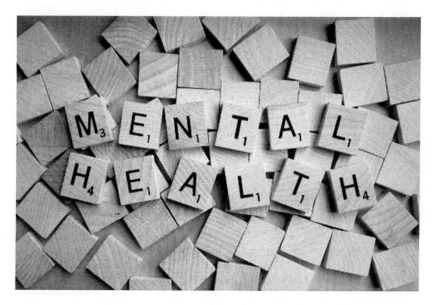

Mental health

Memory is how we speak of who we are and what makes us. It is hard to picture one day that we won't be able to access those moments.

Forgetting is one ordinary occurrence that all of us experience at least once in our lives. This issue may not be something of our intention, but is a natural manifestation that grows with our age.

Memory loss (amnesia) has been one of the hottest elements in Asian Drama TV series in which someone gets a bump on the head and wakes up aimlessly. This profound memory loss is unusual in reality, but is brought onto the show to gain audiences.

However, the variant of it is a real problem.

In a flashback, remember how many times you misplaced your house keys or when what you just told yourself to do went completely away from your mind?

To some degree, these are a sign of memory loss, but not on the severe side. People forget things and never take it for granted when they are young.

In general, there are two factors involved in causing this shortcoming of brain; namely heredity and life events.

While genetics is an inevitable risk factor, the way you treat your health also plays a critical role.

Our mortality includes a great number of downsides. Forgetfulness is a sign of brain defects. The consequence relates to many aspects that can be kept in our control in our younger days like medical conditions, diet, and lifestyle.

But most of us prefer enjoying our lives with less consciousness toward dementia. That may bring some regrets when you reach the other half of the path. As a result of aging and treatable conditions, many will develop Alzheimer's disease and related disorders.

Imagine you can't remember the name of your son and grandchild; you don't know if you need a bathroom break and are unsure about what is going on when people are celebrating Christmas. Isn't that sad?

But growing old doesn't have to come with such suffering. Don't live through the rest of your time with such irritation while there exists methods to block dementia.

That said, it is crucial to equip yourself with knowledge about the problem and help you to figure out how you can deal with it.

You are not alone in facing this issue. This E-book is created to prevent and cure memory loss problems.

Everything you need to know about memory is here and it also provides the neurobic training you need to exercise your brain.

Getting yourself prepared before the wave of memory loss comes is always better than running when it's already here.

This E-book will help you:

- To identify mild forgetfulness and more serious dementia-related issues
- To learn about memory loss, its causes, signals, and how to treat them
- To exercise your brain before it wears out with age

CHAPTER II: OVERVIEW

Here you are, at the first doorstep to strive against forgetting the beauty of your past. In this chapter, you will go through the definition of memory loss and dig deeper into our brain's mechanism.

More than that, you will know what affects your brain's function, the common causes of the problem, as well as the signs, symptoms, consequences, and everything you need to preserve your battle.

Linda's story

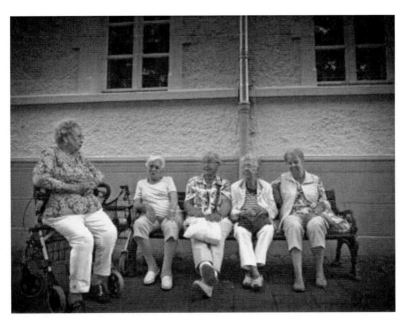

Linda and her friends

At her golden age, Linda finds herself enjoying looking at her grandchildren swimming in the backyard from the porch. But she can't remember the story her grandson told her about the science fair yesterday. When she got to where she had to ask about what her beloved people did the day before, she feels her brain is playing tricks on her. And she can't stop blaming herself for not recalling anything.

In her check-up, the doctor said she had just entered the first stage of dementia, and forgetfulness is a normal part of it. He suggested Linda attend a community center and have fun around memory improving games like playing cards with friends or doing social work. That way, she can find the meaning of life in her time left and boost her brain's health.

A. Memory loss, MCI, and dementia: What's the difference?

When you are unable to retrieve information, there is something damaged in your brain. People will experience a moment when they can't recall an event, a name or even the one they spent time with.

Memory loss is a broad term that can translate into many types of brain malfunctions and amnesia syndrome is a clinical term that infers the initial phase of more critical types of memory impairment.

This health complaint can be temporary or permanent depending on the causes. A variety of young adults in a survey confess that they usually forget where they put their keys, pens and sometimes they even don't know if they turned off the heater. That may due to a heavy workload, being absent-minded, and distraction. But the underlying causes can be worse.

Dementia is the inability of cognitive function. In other words, it is a disorder in which people have difficulty in thinking, retrieving memory and reasoning. These include language skills, self-management, visual perception and defects in many personal skills. You can easily catch a person with dementia losing his/her temperament and changing their personality.

Statics shows up to half of the elderly older than 85 may suffer some forms of dementia and this is not a normal part of aging like mere memory loss.

Unlike memory loss, **Mild Cognitive Impairment (MCI) is** diagnosed in people that have minor problems with verbal or problem-solving skills. However, this form of declined memory is not a form of dementia. Though the signs are noticeable and mistaken for aging, MCI is not serious enough to interfere with daily life.

Concerning **Alzheimer's**, MCI is considered the early stage of the disease. It doesn't always progress to Alzheimer's. Nonetheless, many studies found that approximately 32% of MCI diagnosed is likely to develop into Alzheimer's within 5 years.

1. The role of memory

Needless to say, memory consists of footage of whatever happened to your perception that is recorded and stored in an area of your brain. It gives you knowledge, relationship, feeling and everything you need to live a full life. People without a memory would be unsettled and in extreme fear.

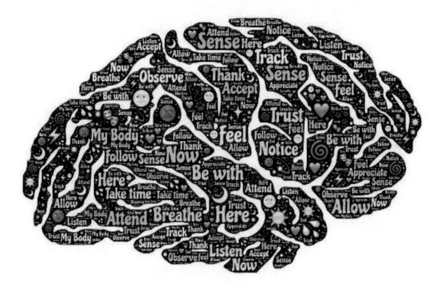

The brain

For example, I am using my memory of the keys on this computer keyboard to type. My brain is searching the section of what I know about the topic to stream my words onto the page. I'm also remembering the experience I have with "memory" to outline, to express my opinion and to write down what you are reading. Memory allows you to manifest the skills you learned, as well as to record and recall your happy moments. Above all, *the past gives you the motivation to move on.*

After all, your memory as a biological planner with data collected from the time you went through that lets you access the right cue when need. Losing memory is worse than a curse, and it's hard to imagine you have to step forward without knowing what made you do so.

Click to follow link to get free bonus:

https://rebrand.ly/memory-cure-book

2. How does your memory function?

Let's take a trip into your brain and see how it retains information.

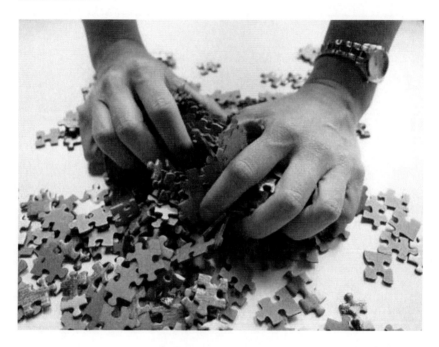

Pieces of memory

Whenever you witness an event, learn a fact or experience something that goes directly to imprint into your mind, some parts of the brain kickstarts the memory crafting process. This occurrence involves plenty of components to trigger the network, which I can name some here: the hippocampus, thalamus, amygdala, putamen, prefrontal cortex, basal ganglia and so on.

Scientifically, your brain records the information and places the pieces into encoding. The member components will be responsible for transmitting the name of a person, the smell of a roasted chicken or the feeling for your crush to the encoded area. If you forget what just happened right after the moment, probably it was not encoded, or because you weren't paying attention.

Now you can remember the piece of data; the next step is to retrieve it when it's time to recall. It is like trying to apply what you learned about minus and subtract to do your homework.

The great thing is every time you remember something, meaning that you bring that piece of information to the neural pathway again and again. This action indeed consolidates the path to make the memory easier to recall. That is how scientists invent activities you can participate in to boost the remembering part of your brain.

3. Types of memory loss, symptoms and causes

In the definition, I have explained memory loss and a few of its variants. In the deeper sea, there are certain types of problems related to brain cells dying that causes memory difficulties. Since the sub-categories are wide, I sorted them out in two major types: Temporary and Permanent. Medically, they are Transient global amnesia and long-term memory loss.

Transient global amnesia

Misplacing household objects, looking for your glasses while you have them in your hand or walking to a room and having no idea why you are there, are all examples of normal temporary memory loss.

With transient global amnesia, middle-aged or old people are unable to form a new memory, but can remember the recent past. Though it is not as bad as not knowing who you are, the sudden forgetfulness can be frightening.

Symptoms

To diagnose transient amnesia, these signs must present:

- Repeatedly asking the same question, not frequently
- Can identify self
- Cognition appears to be normal
- Memory can recover
- No head injury in recent history
- No history of epilepsy

Causes

What leads to temporary memory loss depends on underlying many factors. The possible cause can lie in the overload of blood veins or a history of migraines. Although the likelihood of those drives is low, there are reported culprits that may ignite the issue. These are:

- Strenuous muscular activity
- Mild head trauma
- Sexual intercourse
- Angiography or endoscopy procedures
- Emotional distress
- Stroke
- Mental Shock

Also, the clearest risk factor is in the age of the individual. Declining brain function due to dead brain cells can happen in the memory, making the process less efficient. Thus, it leads to blackouts and amnesia.

Permanent memory loss

Remember the MCI I mentioned earlier? Long-term memory loss includes impairment and some forms of it. The most obvious sign of this disorder is forgetting events that occurred in early life which you never want to wipe off the memory. Maybe they are the name of your high school, or the date of your wedding anniversary.

Symptoms

Although some people may laugh at you about forgetting your own birthday, long-term memory loss involves something more serious. If you catch yourself (if possible) or your family members experience these signs, you should consult a specialist. These are:

- Verbal confusion, like calling a dog a cat
- Language Difficulty
- Get lost in a familiar neighborhood
- Take a long time to complete a task
- Personality change
- Become grumpier

Causes

The natural causes may originate from a deficiency of genetics or a brain tumor. But there are reversible factors that can be treated if one is aware of his condition when he grows old. These are:

- Depression
- Medication affect
- Misuse of alcohol and drug
- Brain injuries
- Epilepsy
- Brain infection

If the impairment develops into dementia or Alzheimer's, it is beyond the current remedy.

Remember that dementia can cause memory loss, but long-term or short-term memory impairment doesn't have to lead to dementia. But whatever is it, what happens at the end is an irritation that leads to many changes in one person.

4. Reversible causes

I have mentioned about treatable causes that can be handled by the individuals. Upon the current medical use of a patient, doctors can screen for the conditions and make recommendations to reverse the causes. The possible reversible causes of memory loss include:

- Emotional disorder: Anxiety, stress, shock, or depression
- Vitamin B-12 deficiency: Lack of nerve cell and red blood cell feeder
- Minor head trauma: Head injury from an accident
- Medications: One medication or a combination of drugs
- Alcoholism: Chronic disorder
- Hypothyroidism: An underactive thyroid gland
- Brain diseases: Brain tumor or infection

5. The consequences of memory loss

Both temporary and permanent memory loss can interfere with your daily life. People with memory problems find it hard to store recent events and conversations. How frustrating would it be if you can't recall what you talked about yesterday with your colleague? Do you see the risk of losing the plot of the meeting and a fat contract? What if you forget to lock the apartment door and lost all your valuables in one morning?

Permanent memory loss brings even more desperation. The fragments in your memory take away your ability to hold a regular conversation. You would feel your intelligence is moving far away. You might not find your way home even if it's only a few miles away.

In the emotional aspect, memory is precious. Forgetting a cherished minded memento is a huge loss. People in late adolescence or elderly adulthood with dementia can recall significant moments or events that repeat in a high frequency. Their brains may imprint some certain dates with an emotional influence so that the strong emotions will remind them of the facts. Think about September 11, 2001; people are likely to connect to the flashback of where they were at that time.

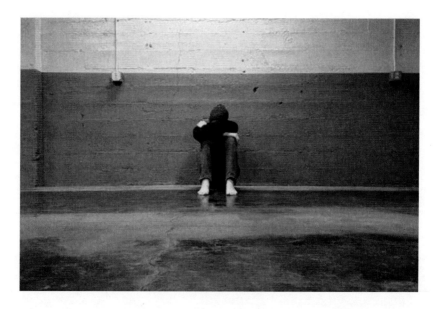

No clue

Although the familiarity still lodges in the subconscious, what is left in the mind is only a vaporous picture that leaves uncertain feelings. Such emotion is pretty full of anxiety. Therefore, it is understandable why individuals with memory impairments are typically uneasy and out of sorts.

If the matter does not receive prompt treatment, the worst thing memory loss can lead to should be Alzheimer's. Alzheimer's patients face a number of health declines, including mindful impairments. The disease starts with misplacing common objects, keeping wondering about one thing, or forgetting the eaten meals. In the severe stage, the person may not be able to walk, ask for food or function on a daily basis.

Worse, the patient may piss himself, fall off on the floor causing other trauma, or get lost. Some cases forward to their death due to malnutrition because they are unable to call when hungry, or of infected injuries that the patient doesn't remember to tell the family about.

The consequences of memory loss can be heart-rending. The help from family and society is exceptionally crucial for people with memory loss at any stage. Don't let the situation get worse when there is still a way to save it. Try to support and assist the sick person with all the means you can afford.

B. How dementia relates to alzheimer's

The relationship between dementia and Alzheimer's is apparently close. While dementia is a general term covering a group of symptoms affecting the mental cognition, Alzheimer's is a disease under the "umbrella" of dementia.

Since dementia includes Alzheimer's in its diagnosed syndromes, people who get informed of having any memory impairment face a higher risk of it developing into the brain disease.

1. Risk factors

Although the causes are still under researches, there are a couple of factors that contribute to the chance of getting Alzheimer's. These are:

- **Age**: One study shows that per 1,000 elderlies from 65 to 85, around 5% will get diagnosed with the disease.
- **Down syndrome:** Researchers explain the relation as in the creation of beta-amyloid that leaves toxic fragments to affect the neurons. Down syndrome patients can develop Alzheimer's 10 to 20 years earlier.
- **Genetics and family history:** The trigger may lie in rare mutations passed from the previous generation which account for less than 1%, but guarantee Alzheimer's.
- **MCI:** Those who got informed of MCI may become aware of the situation and begin to compensate for memory loss by consulting medical help.

- **Heart health:** People with obesity, high blood pressure, high cholesterol or diabetes type 2 face a greater chance of developing Alzheimer's.

2. Would any form of dementia lead to Alzheimer's disease?

The understanding of the causes of Alzheimer's remains elusive. Scientists believe it has something to do with the gene and its combination. Lifestyle and outside factors also contribute to the defects of the brain over time.

Alzheimer's and brain

When brain proteins fail to function, it damages neurons and leads to disruption of these brain cells. Consequently, the dead component unleashes toxin to kill its surrounding habitats. This process may happen years before the first symptoms appear. The occurrence often takes place in the brain part that controls memory, then spreads until the brain gets wholly shrunk.

Plaques, tangles, and their roles

According to the autopsy studies, plaques and tangles grow with age, even more rapidly in those with Alzheimer's potent. It is still unexplainable how these structures are the prime suspects in the destruction of nerve cells, but many believe they block the communication among these cells.

Understanding the reason behind Alzheimer's, we can see the relationship between the two terms is clear. Alzheimer's, as a cause of dementia, is considered the final stage of any diagnosed memory impairment. The involvement counts other elements as risks. That said, any deficiency in the brain's function poses all the likelihood of one person getting the disease of Alzheimer's.

C. Prevent and cure

There is no existence of a medical cure for memory loss of all types. The best bet at the moment is blocking its way when there is still time. Lifestyle is one crucial key to have a healthy body and mind when you get old. But the reversible causes are what you can actually bring under control.

Seeing a doctor is a must and it's the first thing you should do if the symptoms are around. A set of questions will be made to diagnose the issue. Those can include:

- When did you first feel the memory malfunctions?
- Have you had a recent accident?
- Did it hurt anything on or close to the head?
- What is in your current prescription?
- Are you on a diet? What are the supplements you're taking?
- Do you feel anxious, depressed, or just sad?
- Do you find any task difficult?
- How much alcohol do you have a day?
- Have you recently started a new drug?
- Are you experiencing any notable loss or change in your life?

Coming after the questions would be a physical exam. Your doctor may also conduct a blood test and brain-imaging tests to identify the causes. Then, he can be able to give pieces of advice.

Although pills at the moment can't swap the condition

magically, they can lessen the impairments. Moreover, a healthy way of living and diet can contribute enhancements to a growing-old brain.

In all circumstances, a combination of moderate medication use and a wholesome lifestyle is a perfect prevention from dementia.

1. Medication treatment

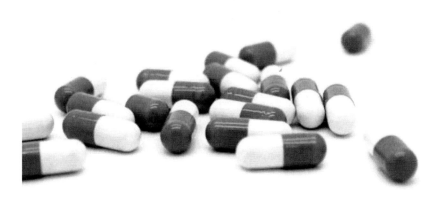

Medications

The U.S. Food and Drug Administration, aka FDA, has approved the effectiveness of two types of medications to treat memory impairments and its variations including symptoms of Alzheimer's disease. Those are Cholinesterase Inhibitors from Exelon, Aricept, Razadyne and Memantine from Namenda. The newest medical release is Namzaric, whose formula is from the previous two types.

These medicines help to mask the symptoms, and blind them to steer toward your brain, - not eliminate or delay cell damage.

Here is a table of treatments-at-a-glance:

Generic	Brand	FDA-Approval year	Stage severity	Side Effects
Donepezil	Aricept	1996	All stages	Nausea, vomiting, appetite deficiency and increased frequency of bowel movements.
Galantamine	Razadyne	2001	Mild to moderate	Nausea, vomiting, appetite deficiency and increased frequency of bowel movements.
Rivastigmine	Exelon	2000	Mild to moderate	Nausea, vomiting, appetite deficiency and increased frequency of bowel

				movements.
Memanti ne	Name nda	2003	Moder ate to severe	Headache, dizziness, constipation, and confusion.
Memanti ne + Donepezi l	Namza ric	2014	Moder ate to severe	Nausea, vomiting, loss of appetite, increased the frequency of bowel movements, headache, constipation, confusion, and dizziness.

Reference:

https://www.alz.org/alzheimers-dementia/treatments/medications-for-memory

https://thecrcnj.com/medication-memory-impairment-2/

Cholinesterase inhibitors

For light to moderate stages, a member of these generics including Donepezil, Rivastigmine, and Galantamine will be responsible. Cholinesterase inhibitors stop the cholinesterase enzyme from wiping acetylcholine off the synapses, or the gap between neurons. It also prevents this organic chemical messenger from breaking down, keeping it high to support the connection among nerve cells. With acetylcholine maintained in the brain, it preserves memory function more effectively for learning, memorizing and boosting mood.

Furthermore, the inhibitor slows down the worsening of symptoms. However, it includes a low side-effect profile varied from person to person.

Memantine

This NMDA receptor antagonist is a mixture of donepezil and memantine. It modulates the activity of the information processing chemical called glutamate and prevents the intruding of calcium into the neurons that can cause a cascade of damage. Its modest benefit offers an improvement in mental health and the capability to practice daily activities.

Effectiveness and side effects precautions

You can expect the medicine to stun the symptoms for a while, but they can't block the underlying disease process of plaque or untangle parts of the mess. Even with the use of medications, the signs continue to progress. Side effects, fortunately, are less common. But if anything, those include agitation, drowsiness, constipation, tremors, headaches, fatigue, nausea and insomnia. Memantine, on the contrary, it can result in sleepiness.

2. Eating right

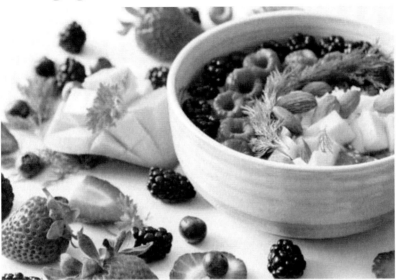

Healthy diet

A nourishing diet impacts significantly on both physical and mental health. Since the brain is the management center of the whole body, it is a big deal to feed it the right food so that the control can stay stable.

Research published by Harvard medical school confirms the connection between the diet and memory via a study conducted at Brigham and Women's hospital.

Evidence shows that saturated fats from red meat and butter contribute to building up Low-density lipoprotein (LDL) cholesterol that imperils arteries.

"We know that's bad for your heart. There is now a lot of evidence that it's also bad for your brain."

Dr. Francine Grodstein

Although the exact reason for this linking of saturated fats and poor memory remains unclear, it may relate to apolipoprotein E gene, or APOE. People who have APOE e4, a variation of APOE, are facing a higher risk for Alzheimer's.

"About 65% of individuals who wind up with dementia due to Alzheimer's disease in their 60s and 70s have that gene."

Dr. Gad Marshall

Regardless of the brilliant concept, how the APOE a4 influences dementia is still something waiting to be discovered.

Nevertheless, we know there is a way to swap the condition relying on our meals. Take the Mediterranean diet for example. The components are said to promote brain health. Those include vegetables, whole grains, yogurt, fish, fruit and olive oil. Moderate consumption of alcohol is also a plus to raise healthy LDL levels.

Many doctors claim that **what's good for the heart can be heroes for the mind** too. In the relationship of unclogged blood vessels suffice oxygen for brain cells to deprive, it is a vital need to protect the heart to preserve the brain.

Fish

Being a rich source of Omega-3 fatty acids, fish is always in the list of every food recommendation for the brain. Why? Because 60% of your brain is made of fat in which half of that fat is the Omega-3 kind. This type of fat is vital for building up nerve cells.

The docosahexaenoic acid, or popularly known as DHA, is an essential attribute for normal functioning of neurons establishing your learning and memorizing ability.

A study found that those who ate baked and broiled fish regularly have more gray matter. This component plays a major key in controlling your emotion, and decision making skills.

You should eat:

Salmon, mackerel, tuna, or any fatty fish that is rich in Omega-3 fatty acids.

Berries

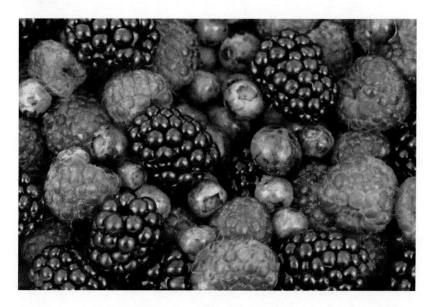

Berries

Berries in a deep color are a host of numerous health benefits targeting your brain. They provide anthocyanins, a group of plant compounds responsible for anti-inflammatory and antioxidant effects. The antioxidants strive against oxidative stress and inflammation, which are the main culprits of brain aging and neurodegenerative disease.

This superfood is moreover reputable for boosting cognitive function even in old age. In a recent study, an experiment showed that healthy elderly from 65 to 70 who drank 30 milliliters of blueberry juice had gained a decent improvement in brain activity.

Thanks to the high content of flavonoids, blueberries are proven to delay the aging process while stimulating blood flow and oxygen to the brain. At Reading University in 2009, an experiment found participants who drank a blueberries smoothie every morning could perform better in concentrating than the ones who didn't.

A 2016 study also demonstrated eating blueberries can reduce the genetic and biochemical radicals behind anxiety and suicidal tendencies. And tons of health benefits are obtained from this tasty fruit. Make sure you talk to your doctor before starting consuming blueberries for memory treatment.

Click to follow link to get free bonus:

https://rebrand.ly/memory-cure-book

Avocado

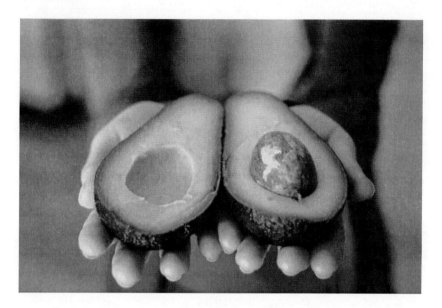

Avocado

The creamy treat contains a myriad of Vitamin E and C that is proved to rock your brain. Besides, avocado has loads of healthy fats that are beneficial for feel-good mood and emotion. The Omega-3 fatty acids in this fruit aid in cholesterol reduction and help your body to absorb nutrients.

Theory says, "A healthy flow means a healthy brain," the monounsaturated fat in avocado is a huge dedication to seamless blood flow. It also lowers blood pressure and that reduces the risk factor for hypertension. However, avocado is high in calories. That means you need to pay attention to using it in a scientific fashion. One-fourth to a half a day is an ideal amount for your brain and entire body.

Eggs

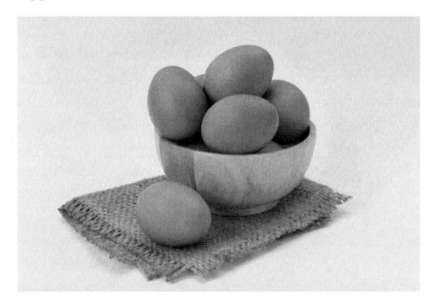

Egg

There are countless benefits of eggs to our health system, including the mind. Eggs are full of vitamin B6, B12, folate, and choline that are tied to brain health. If you recall the role of the neurotransmitter acetylcholine in promoting memory, it is formulated with choline as a micronutrient.

Choline has a major function in regulating mood and memory. The constituent presents mostly in egg yolk, which everyone can add to their daily meal. An adequate intake of choline ranges from 425mg to 550mg per day depending on gender and body condition.

Folate and B12 have several roles in managing depression.

Studies have shown that folic acid is involved in the mental declining process. It minimizes senescence. B12 is responsible for synthesizing brain chemicals and keeps the sugar levels in the brain stable.

Other natural antioxidant sources

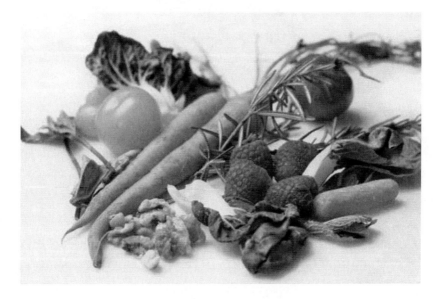

Fruits contain antioxidants

Turmeric, pumpkin seeds, and broccoli are wholesome contributors of antioxidants. In broccoli, they found a high concentration of the fat-soluble vitamin K, which is essential for forming sphingolipids which have a dense population in brain cells.

The active ingredient curcumin in turmeric can help clear the amyloid plaques to improve the memory of Alzheimer's patients. Furthermore, the compound increases the amount of serotonin and dopamine to fight against depression.

Pumpkin seeds are an excellent source of magnesium, copper, zinc, and iron. Those elements are crucial for the nerve mechanism and should be served to prevent multiple brain malfunctions.

Besides, caffeine, flavonoids, and antioxidants in dark chocolate are all legit brain-food. In a 900-people conduction, those who consumed dark chocolate were found to perform more efficiently in various mental tasks than the ones who ate crackers.

Those are just a few in the endless line of things you can eat for the brain. There are more common foods present in the grocery store that are friends of the memory network than you think.

Have a look at this Food for Memory chart:

Food Name	Nutrient Brain Values	Effect
Tomatoes	Lycopene antioxidant	Prevent free radical damage
Citrus fruits (Orange, broccoli,	Vitamin C	Increase mental agility

blackcurrant,…)		
Sage (Salvia)	Phenolic acids and flavonoids	Boost memory and concentration
Beets, Celery, Cabbage, Spinach.	Nitrates Endothelial NO	Aid vascular to transfer oxygen to the brain
Vegetable Oil (Olive Oil, Coconut Oil)	Natural anti-inflammatory	Improve learning and memory
Nuts (peanuts, walnuts, hazelnut,…)	Healthy Fats Antioxidants Vitamin E Omega-3 (walnuts)	Protect healthy brain function

3. Lifestyle change

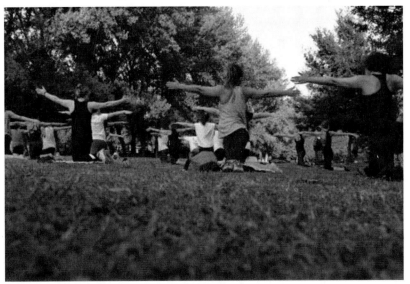

Healthy lifestyle

A healthy way of living benefits the entire body, not only the brain. The better you take care of yourself, the better your brain is likely to be.

Doctors at NYU Langone Healthy emphasize the importance of staying physically active in keeping the mind engaged. Mainly, regular aerobic exercise can actually slow the cognitive decline.

Diet is a part of a memory-improving pattern. Consuming such foods as in the list above is a perfect way to protect your cognitive system. Maintaining a healthy diet can also decrease the chance of catching heart disease.

Forgetfulness and MCI are results of overusing alcohol. Cutting back on drinking will leave a significant change affecting the brain, metabolism and reduce the risks of getting diabetes.

Smoking is a huge villain to the body as a whole. Nicotine damages the blood vessels and heart, causing blockages that prevent oxygen from traveling to the brain, thus suffocating the memory network. To the brain, it kills nerve cells leaving defects after a short time using tobacco. The peril in smoking is long-term and fatal. Stopping smoking is the one top priority anyone who wants to thrive against memory loss has to practice immediately.

Doctors encourage staying active in society to stimulate mental health. Communication is a healthy activity to keep people socialized. The act of chatting and sharing is an imperative need that can maintain a high stage of satisfaction. Frequent social interactions also enriches cognitive function in aging people.

Participation in a social community is a positive way of living. People can attend a reading group, or play board games, cards, or a musical instrument to exercise the mind and get engaged with society.

Staying organized is one great tip to make the brain work. Practice jotting down tasks and appointments in your notebook. Group the documents into categories. Separate small bills and large bills in your wallet. Organize spices in the cupboards. Those are tasks that help connect what you retain and you can have fast access to them. This way also limits distractions and leaves you time to retrieve the exact information you need.

Having a good sleep is a key factor in perfect health. Needless to say, knowing how insomnia terrorizes nerve cells and memory system, it is a must to give yourself a nice rest as well as letting the brain sleep. 8-hours is the ideal time range for full body relaxation.

After all, the means for having a lucid mind has everything to do with healthy blood flow and the heart. The idea of keeping your brain sound is to keep all medical conditions under control. People with chronic illnesses like high blood pressure, depression, high blood cholesterol, obesity, and diabetes have all the likelihood to develop dementia. Therefore, it is crucial to manage those health issues. It is best to review your medications with your physician or psychiatrist.

4. Meditations to mindwork

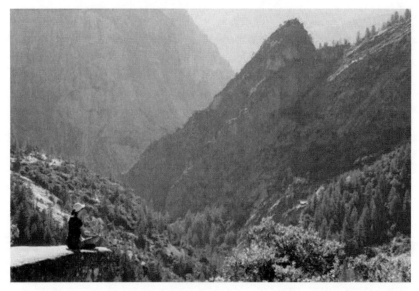

Meditation

There is no doubt about the far-reaching benefits of meditation. Neuroscientists have confirmed in several studies about the connection of this peaceful activity and memory enhancement. In Boston, researchers conducted an investigation and learned that meditation appears to fortify the cerebral cortex that handles mental abilities like learning and focusing.

The basic idea is sitting still with a floating mind helps pump blood to the brain, which consolidates the blood vessel network.

"Meditation training can enhance various cognitive processes, such as emotional regulation, executive control, and attention, particularly sustained attention."

Social Cognitive and Affective Neuroscience Journal

Bingo! This is even more natural and easier than keeping a diet. Virtually anyone can take these techniques into practice and enjoy the benefits.

The most relevant target in meditation is to get a high stage of concentration. This attentional control is an element for creating a complete memory. The more extended this span is, the broader the capacity of your short-term waiting room becomes.

Observations indicate experienced Buddhist monks are the best practitioner of meditation. Although the biological mechanisms behind this method are quite a mystery, its evidence is incontestable. Good news is, you don't have to be a monk to meditate.

5. Mistakes that will sabotage your memory

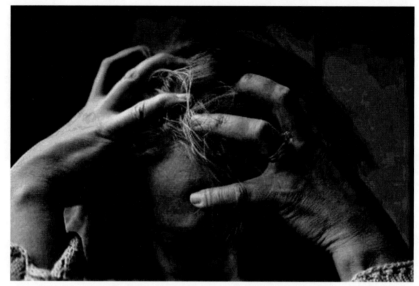

Depression and confusion

In treating your short-term memory, chances are you will keep up with your mental to-do list and rest assured you will never forget practicing on the next presentation that dues in 2 days. Worse, a brilliant idea popped out in your mind, but slipped out just as quick as the way it came.

The thing is that your short-term memory is finite. Recent studies show that the brain can hold on average four pieces of information in the short-term storage. You can figure it like holding FOUR coconuts in two hands. That leaves no room for the fifth one; so if you are too stubborn and you want to add one more coconut, another one will fall off your hand. That's how you lose a piece of memory.

If the short-term memory is an overcrowded waiting room, long-term memory is one of endless storage. When the piece of short-term memory gets encoded, it becomes a long-term memory. And the place for long-term guests is unlimited. However, it can squeeze down with age and you can drop every piece of memory if a person enters the memory loss stage.

Aside from attempting to boost your memory, you may make the mistake of stuffing it. You are likely to keep the information waiting to be processed in the room rather than actually wielding it. You can blame that constant stream of Facebook notifications for overloading your storage. But be aware that the room is bubbling up and the nerve staff has no way to handle the crowd. That is when you fail the system.

Another interesting side effect of practicing reinforcing memory is people tend to strengthen and rehearse failure. Admittedly, this bizarre habit happens when your mistake comes along with fear. You may demand your inner self not to repeat that mistake, but you get more success than failure in duplicating the same wrong.

I recall the first time I got into trouble remembering the names of members in my favorite music band. I feared people would taunt me for being a dumb fan. Although with all the hard work to remember all 6 of them, I failed like ten times retrieving their names, not to mention their faces.

In the end, I figured out how to attach a silly picture to each of them with each name sketching out like the running lyrics in karaoke. Sure enough, I encoded the images rather than the letters, though the letter itself is a form of perception.

This explains the way our memory perceives the trash data. We follow the pattern that impresses us the most with emotion and make it a long-term memory.

The challenge of not taxing your short-term is nothing but learning how to stop cramming in details and unclogging the unfinished tasks. Also, short-term memory can increase its capacity if you practice the right exercises. That said, decluttering your short-term memory, fortunately, has a method to follow.

Take advantage of technology by using task managing platforms like Evernote, or just a plain paper planner. Make a list of everything you need to accomplish, include the all the details. The list is your secondary warehouse that will remind you of the tasks once you review it. You can add more information if needed.

After all, when you find yourself floundering, probably the short-term storage is flooded. Take time to meditate, breath, and release the string in your mind.

6. Coping strategies for memory loss to practice daily

Memory loss wipes little details off your mind. It would be a misery if people didn't find a way to overcome their forgetfulness. In reality, it is possible to improve the function of the brain if you can wake it up from the sluggish stage. Science has found that a small practice every day helps consolidate your general memory capacity. For people with symptoms of memory loss, besides reinforcing the mind with diet, change of lifestyle, meditation, and medicine, they can get support from their surroundings.

Here are various activities you can stuff the reminders to potential forgettable subjects in your everyday life, or utilize natural memory aids to get along with the impairment.

Everyday life

Making a routine

Forming a habit helps imprint a pattern into your brain. Repeating a certain sequence makes it a long-term memory that you can easily retrieve because the recurrence has implanted an unconscious reaction towards one deed. You can develop a routine for everything and train your mind to become an autopilot. It is able to walk you through what is there in the line every day.

You can start by doing things in order. For example, organize your purse in the same manner. You will put the keychain in first, then a lipstick, tissues, charger then some cash at the end. Always place these items in the same position where you can find them.

Doing things in order will remind you what comes after one task. If you wash the dishes after dinner, then vacuum the living room, prepare your suitcase for work tomorrow, then brush the teeth and go to bed, that same sequence can help you recall what's missing.

One thing once

Don't attempt multitasking because your short-term memory has a limited capacity. Memory loss has further squeezed down the size of this waiting room. So, the best thing you should do is to focus on one job at a time. You've got your reminder to retrieve; don't push it too hard on your memory.

Things at its positions

You will know where to find your car key in case it is not where it's supposed to be. In the kitchen, for example, the pan should be hung above the counter, knives and forks are in the drawer. You can get access quickly to these items without needing to probe your memory.

Memorize numbers

What I do when I need to memorize a phone number is I make a rhyme out of it. But if you're not confident with your musical skill, you can write or visualize how the numbers typed are on a keypad. Making an association is also a great tip. You can connect the number 8 with "Ate," 1 with "want," 4 with "for," and so on. Try to picture the sequence with humor. An exaggerated image is always easier to remember.

Automatic payment

Technology allows you to pay a bill automatically once it gets announced. Add a credit card and set an auto payment.

Secure important paper in one place

If you have a wall safe, or any one place to store all your work documents, gather them all in that place. Make sure you don't create a new mess.

Think about speaking to your solicitor

You should think about if you need to talk to your solicitor to put your affairs in order.

Pill boxes

A pillbox with divided slots helps you take the right medicine in time. Split your prescription into days then add to each slot. Leave the box somewhere obvious.

Memory Aids

To-do list

A to-do list is a great reminder that helps you memorize your tasks. You may keep one on the fridge, in your pulse and at the front door.

Wallboard or table calendar

Place a table calendar and take advantage of its spaces. A wallboard in your workplace also offers generous room to note down things to do.

Times and dates

You should use a clock, a watch or a calendar to help you keep track of times and dates. You should buy watches that you can set to remind you of things and clocks with large faces.

Notebook

Keep a small notebook with you to quickly write down whatever mission that crosses your day.

Gadget help

The support of cutting-edge gadgets will store the memory for you. Consider them as your external hard drive. To make use of the smart device effectively, you should prioritize the reminder app and make it a habit to use the phone to note a long-term memory.

Timers

It will ring a bell at a set time you want to accomplish a task. Remember to stick the specific job you need to complete on the timers.

Be social

Name printing

Verbalize the name instead of mentally noting it. Sounding out the name (not shouting) can imprint its impression in your mind way more effectively. Or you can associate the name with someone with a similar name you know. If the person is Harry, you can associate it with Harold or Henry. Unless the name is unusual or you don't know anyone with the same name, make a mental note.

Give yourself a break

Don't push yourself too hard on remembering things. Stress is the enemy to the brain, hence to you. You've got all the help from people to technology. More importantly, don't feel embarrassed if you can't retrieve your memory.

Advice for the brain's well-being

Getting a health check-up should always be your priority. Pieces of advice from doctors and experts are valuable in any aspect. Thus, get routine health checks every once in a while to keep yourself, as well as your brain, in optimal condition.

D. Help someone with memory impairments

The first and foremost thing anyone should do when one suspects abnormal signs in memory function is to visit a doctor. If that person is your family member, help him/her to book an appointment.

Here is the check-list of the symptoms:

- Asking the same questions again and again
- Having difficulty in conversation
- Misplacing items
- Getting lost
- Forgetting common words
- Changing in mood and behavior
- Becoming more aggressive, grumpier

To some degree, people don't take the signs seriously until severity becomes notable. Especially to the elderly, the necessity of medical help is in prior. Dementia has three stages, that doesn't mean people can wait until the last moment to get treatment. Wouldn't it be better if the sickness is caught in its hatching phase?

The situation may get worse if you recognize these signs:

- Forgetfulness becomes more persistent
- Increase the frequency of repeating the same questions
- Have trouble walking
- Forget an important name
- Exposed to have any sign of Alzheimer's

These mindful changes should not be ignored. Memory loss is not lethal, but it causes aches in emotion and makes people suffer every day. Although some forms of dementia are a normal part of aging, we don't want our loved ones to tolerate this irritation in their left time.

Seeing someone forgetting his name is not ridiculous. Consider that as one sign of early dementia, and there are particular things you can do to help. Your care comes in critical in this case.

1. What can a family do to help?

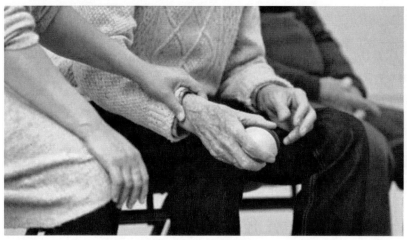

Family help

If you have a memory impairment patient at home, your duty is to help the person maintain his independence, confidence, and dignity as long as possible. These tips may assist you.

Be patient

It is requisite to be forbearing with a forgetful person. They have already lost their blessed mind; they can't afford to lose your sympathy. You don't have to show off your compassion, but specific care speaks a thousand words. Things like answering one question several times without getting upset, reminding the person to do the same task every day, or noticing what the sick one usually forgets and writing down notes in the toilet, kitchen or bedroom.

Be calm

People with dementia lose their confidence in facing trouble. They're conscious of their being a burden, which can downgrade their mood. That directs them to become uneasy and uncomfortable around people. They are likely to isolate themselves and yell at others. Don't take this personal because you know why they are doing it. Sick people can be unreasonable, but they don't want to be that way.

Keep things simple

Take it slow and give the sick people time to adapt to the condition. When reminding them of a task, you want to keep it simple and free of distraction; you can keep repeating and break it down into small steps.

Don't ask questions, but create simple verbal cues. Don't mix up language and use complicated vocabularies.

Make a routine

Too much variety around the house can be confusing to the ill people. You can establish a routine and get the sick familiarized with it. This helps the person feel more secure and follow the right pattern.

2. What can a caregiver do to help?

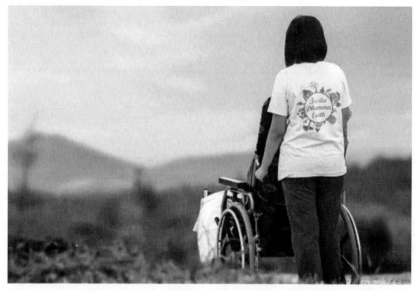

Caregiver help

Your specialty tells you what to do what there are still unexpected things happening. Solving them is a skill to learn. Here are a few tips you can take advantage of.

Communicate right

You are the one who will spend time with the patient, so don't leave the moment empty. As socializing is one of natural treatment, it makes sense to hold conversations. And before entering a chat, let's do a mindset.

Speak in a pleasant and respectful manner. Convey your messages in facial expressions, with a low tone of voice and a gentle touch.

To get attention from the person, reduce the distractions like TV or the surroundings. Introduce yourself, then help the person identify herself, state your name, your role, relation and why you are there. Maintain eye contact.

Deliver your message clearly in a reassuring voice. Take time to repeat the same thing in the same manner; you may want to stress but don't get aggressive. If the person still doesn't get it, you can wait a few minutes, then rephrase what you said. Don't make the sentences complex. The best that works is YES/NO questions. Combine that with showing the choices to make your question more clarified.

When you get the answer, respond with affection. If the feedback is negative, never try to convince the sick that they are wrong. Wait for them to demonstrate their uncertainty and express your compassion. Your attitude should come with physical reassurance to show support. Things like a hug, holding hands, and praise helps a lot in comforting when all attempts fail.

A sense of humor is one factor that eases the situation. Laughter is the best medicine though it's not at the person's expense. However, it helps them retain social skills and trigger their liveliness.

Behave right

The ground rule is that you can't change the person. The brain disorder has shaped the person, and there is no way you can computerize the brain. So, this is not the land to control.

If your patient insists on sleeping on the floor, you can follow and support by placing a mattress on the floor. People with dementia always feel insecure, and disagreeing with them only makes them feel like blowing up. In this case, it is your behavior and the physical environment that you can change.

You can check with the doctor if the behavioral problem keeps on. Perhaps there are some underlying causes due to their medications. Be cautious that people with memory loss can't tell you what they want. For example, they mess up their room looking for nothing, and they do not due it on purpose to piss you off, but to keep themselves productive. You should accommodate the behavior and figure out their wish through time.

The natural progression of the disease process doesn't stay in one place. That means your routine may not work tomorrow or may no longer work at all. This is when your creativity and flexibility come in handy. Sketch up a strategy to deal with the change. By expecting that your patient will have more hard times than good ones, you can always get support and advice from the community.

CHAPTER III: 50 UNCOMMON NEUROBIC EXERCISES TO WAKE UP YOUR BRAIN

We all acknowledge the advantage of staying physically active in the mind. But how to practice the activities in a scientific fashion requires skill. The most recent discovery in neurobiology believes the spontaneous growth of neurotrophin factors can fight off mental aging.

This brilliant concept involves the term "neroubics", which I can easily explain as a mix of neuro and aerobics.

The idea focuses on using five senses – sight, sound, smell, taste, and touch combined with emotion to creat new unique ways to shake up the brain. With the 6 senses in hand, you are able to build a boulevard of six lanes wide enough to load information traffic.

The idea repudiates a view in repeating a task over and over. Neurobics says this is no longer true.

While most of us make use of only seeing and hearing, many pieces of data can't drive the brain toll booth if the section closes due to overloading. As you can involve all senses to open FOUR more lanes, the mental traffic jam becomes smoother.

Now you need an extraordinary way

Follow these 50 neurobic exercises; you will be able to upgrade your waiting house's capacity and keep your memory sharp and young.

A. Touch

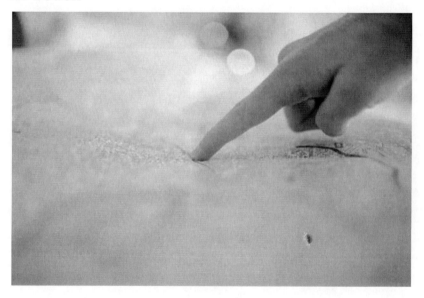

Touch

1. Coin guess

Hide a coin in your pocket or a purse. Then, reach for the coin with your hand and don't let yourself see it. Touch and feel the shape, material, pattern of the coin. Try to figure out which coin it is, the value and what it is made of. You will see how fun it is.

2. Blind shower

The texture of your body that you never felt before will gain attention from your mind. Use your tactile senses to feel, and wash your body while shutting your eyes.

3. Finger gym

There are studies indicating that each fingertip possesses more than 3,000 sensory receptors, which act as a highway to your brain.

Start with inhaling deeply, then bend your elbows and lift your fingers to eye level. Face the palms to each other and let your fingers touch each other. Breath out and lower the right at the same time while folding the left-hand fingers to cover the fingertips of the right hand. It should look like you are catching your right hand sliding down.

Now breath again through your nose and straighten the fingers on your left hand. Simultaneously, move the right palm up and cover the fingertips of the other hand in the same manner as you did with the left hand.

Repeat this exercise 15 times. There is no need to hurry, but try to coordinate your movements and breathing.

4. Finger gym 2

While breathing in and out in a rhythm, lift both arms bent at the elbows facing your mouth. Your pinky fingers should be touching. Clear your lungs with a complete breath out, then hold it like that. After that, inhale through the nose, meanwhile folding all your fingers one-by-one. Do it in the same fashion when unfolding. Repeat this moment at least 10 times.

5. Speeding typing

Typing with 10 fingers in a skill to learn to enjoy the fun out of a computer. Not only are you surfing the keyboard with all fingers, but you also have to remember positions of over a hundred keys so that you don't have to hunt and peck.

A more advanced typing challenge is keyboarding without even looking at the device. Well! Challenge accepted.

6. Wardrobe puzzle

Have someone layout your closet. Close your eyes and use only tactile associations to sort out types of cloth. This exercise helps you practice retrieving information from your memory. Among the things you bought, you know the characteristics and will rely on those to distinguish items.

7. Eye-shut vehicle start

Open your car door with your eyes closed, then slide into the seat. Use only the sense of touch to find the right car key, insert to the keyhole, buckle the seatbelt, then turn on the car's ignition. Make it harder by using this sense of touch and spatial memory to locate the navigator control or button for windshield wipers. When you're all set, drive with both eyes wide open.

8. Blind assemble

Get a model figure and detach the pieces, then place them on a table. Cover your eyes and use only your hands to put them together.

9. Hand reading

If you can manage to get a book for the blind, learn how to read it with your hands, the usual reading method for the visual impaired. The Braille will give you an entirely new challenge that is more than interesting.

B. Smell

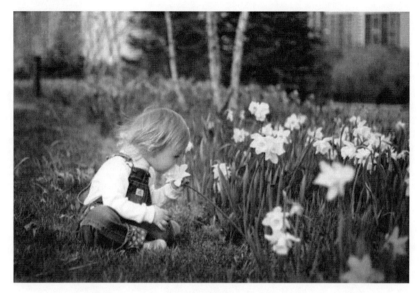

Smell

1. Spice tester

Prepare a bunch of different spices from 10 to 15 ones consisting of parsley, pepper, thyme, oregano, cloves, etc. Close your eyes and smell each jar. Your brain has never experienced this, and it's willing to engage your sense of smell in the new activity.

2. Vanilla wake up

Instead of smelling brewed coffee as you do every usual morning, give your brain a fresh taste from something different. Vanilla is an example. You can also pick other smells like pepper (beware of sneezing), orange, or any kind of herb.

By starting your day with an unusual morning olfactory association of new odor, your neural pathways will respond with positive activation.

3. Smell the world

Maybe you know Hannibal Lecture; he is a genius of olfaction (and killing.) And you see what a brand he's got. You can sharpen your nose by closing the eyes, use only the nose to identify smells around you. You may do this while on the road, in the park or anywhere you find it safe to have your eyes shut.

4. Inhale odorous scent

A strong aroma has a direct influence on the hippocampus, which affects the neural network. This is more like therapy, but you can do it differently by sniffing the essential organic oils such as peppermint, lemon, cinnamon, and citrus. Have a collection of oils and try different scents every day, thus giving your brain a non-routine smelling reinforcement.

C. See

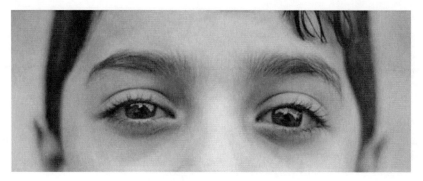

See

1. Make the world slant

Described by Betty Edwards in Drawing on the Right Side of the Brain, looking at non-right-side-up objects triggers the right brain, which is responsible for non-verbal data processing. You can turn over the pictures on the fridge, flip over the clock, or read a note when it's in the wrong way round. This opposite world disables interpreting ability of the "left brain" while activating the "right brain" to awake your sleeping concentration.

2. Supermarket scan

Breaking the routine gives your brain a new task to be busy with. In the exercise, you will enjoy stopping at every aisle in the store, pick up a product you've never seen before and skim its ingredients, then think about it. The new experience always benefits your memory waiting room.

3. Pirate build

Seeing the world with one eye is not like it is with both eyes. Wear an eye patch over one eye and build a small Lego model of a robot, car or airplane with the other opened eye. By losing the depth perception, you will have to rely on new cues and sense of touch to put the pieces together.

4. Picture inspector

Skim the details of an abstract picture and deliver your idea of it. It doesn't have to be profound, just give your sight a stimulation.

5. Reading race

Smart people can read fast. That explains how speed reading can ramp up overall brain function and synaptic density.

D. Hear

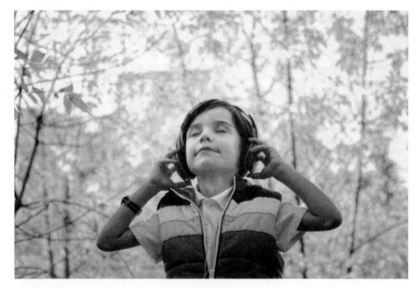

Hear

1. Name that sound

Record sounds from places and put them into a collection. You can gather your family or friends to attend the game. Play the sound and get people to name the sound they hear

2. New music

Don't stick to one genre all day long. Refresh your list by adding new songs of different music. Make it abundant with folk, opera, pop, country, and rock. The new sound will recruit more of the auditory areas, at the same time employ a large scale of neural networks by putting them to work.

3. Read out loud

Reading a text or book out loud will get your sense of hearing in action. The sound gets the brain more engaged than your inner voice. It can promote memorizing and concentration.

4. See with ears

Play a jazz or blues song and try to identify the instrument playing. These genres are rich in the number of instrument attending the band. You will have a variety of answers to work out your brain.

5. Listen to nature

The sound of the wild is endless. Listening to what is shouting out there will freshen up and boost your neural paths. Do this exercise when you're out on vacation. Try to tell what that sound is.

6. Single-ear

Cover up one of your ears and listen with the other to the surrounding sounds. The hearing sense will get up from its comfort zone to pinpoint the sound.

E. Taste

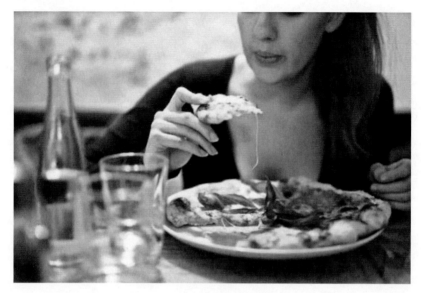

Taste

1. Novel meals

Challenge your taste with a new dinner once in a while. Recording a new taste is like saving your brain's staff from a common job. Since your brain is designed to accept hurdles, new is always better. In this exercise, choose an unusual cuisine and enjoy the fresh seasonings, materials, and freshness.

2. Blind wine tasting

This activity involves at least 3 senses, but your tongue has a major role. Wine experts are capable of distinguishing a different delicacy based on the color, aroma, and taste in wine thanks to the extreme sensitivity of their sense. You can imitate that to the practice.

Try to tell the difference between sweet and sour, heavy and light, sharp and soft. Also, be moderate so as not to lose your balance.

3. Blind dinner

Sounds scary when you don't know what's entering your mouth, but it benefits strengthening your tasting levels. Invite someone to help you do this exercise. Prepare food you never ate before (not the awkward ones). Let your friend feed you randomly while you taste and name the ingredients you can perceive in the recipes.

4. Unknown meal

Collect some spices you never knew about before. Try each of them and depict how it tastes. Recording new savors feeds a job to the nervous system.

5. Novel lunch out

You can experience different cuisine at each meal. It doesn't have to be burgers all day. Make your meal abundant in menus and places.

6. Silent meal

Try not to cause any noise while having your meal and focus on each bite, what makes the taste, and compare it to the last time you had it.

F. Multiple Senses

1. Blind house walking

Close your eyes or put a soft cloth on them and walk around your house. This activity challenges your brain to recall the positions of the objects and furniture in the house. You can walk slowly to avoid falling or kicking items. As you're walking blindly, you are testing your brain on an abnormal routine. That is what neurobics is all about.

2. Dubbing a conversation

You can invite a friend to join this mindful exercise with you. Watch a TV show together, but on mute. You and your pal can invent the contents of the conversation. It is such a great chance to stimulate your brain, as well as showing off your sense of humor.

3. Read out of interest

Get out of the same pattern by reading books on topics you never thought you would touch. For example, don't read more about cars and exotic fashion today. Try the camping guide, or ikebana (Japanese art flower arranging.) New subjects will rouse your creativity and get your brain on a new track.

4. Autopilot drive

Driving following the old map is boring and sleepy to your

mind. Take a new route home to give your brain something out-of-the-way to experience. The new line will get your nervous system engaged and put more effort to attending the fresh test.

5. Awkward writing

I enjoy doing this a lot when I have a chance. You will write with your non-dominant hand. Don't mind the awful letters. It is kind of a rewarding feeling seeing your handwriting improve. It also gives some parts of your brain a job to do.

6. New seat

Experience new seat at every meal to get your brain occupied. You will experience a new position with a new distance to reach the salt, a new view, a different person in front and next to you. Again, NEW is what your brain needs to expand its capacity.

7. Alternative objects

This game helps consolidate your memory retrieving ability. Have a friend hand you an ordinary item, like a book, or a racket. Your mission is to find 10 alternative things, the item can mimic the role. For example, a fly swatter can be a tennis racket, a violin, a boat paddle or a baton.

8. Morning mix-up

Novel tasks are said to shake up a large area of the cortex, that means it can increase brain levels in several distinct areas. Don't make your morning become automatic.

Take a different route to work or change the station. You can try out a kid's program when watching TV. Minor changes won't affect your entire day.

9. Art project

Your nonverbal and emotional parts of the cerebral cortex need an activation. Art is a perfect activity to draw on those and impart new textures. Let your brain go wild on the paper. Be mindless of the outcome.

10. Be social

Holding a conversation is also a great form of brain exercise. Try to be social, proactive. Make friends, talk about things and discover how others think about the world. Receiving new information declutters your brain encoding process.

11. Talk without speaking

In other words, it is learning the Sign language. This moving language requires some of the visual cortex and your hands to display a thought. Sign language integrates several types of sensory information to take part in the communication, thus reinforcing the brain's function. Besides, this is also a rich way to train your sight by reading the idea from the performance and lips of the others.

12. Brain jog

Don't rush to the gym just yet, because the predictable mechanism of the treadmill has nothing to do with your brain. Instead, take it natural into the run. You can go jogging in a park, a trail or cycling off the road. Trying something unpredictable will get your mind to respond to the changes. And don't do the same the next day. Maybe walk with your dog tomorrow, and run to a different neighborhood the day after that.

13. Grow brain garden

You may not believe it, but gardening is one excellent neurobic exercise. You will apply all of your senses to take care of the plants and flowers. Chances are you will smell, touch, look, hear and even taste the seeds or sprigs of herbs. Your brain will plan and urge the spatial abilities to get to business. When all this is incorporated, compensate each other, and your brain will smile.

More than that, the reward is splendid. You'll get fresh, natural and tasty homegrown fruits and vegs, and a beautiful yard too.

14. New hobby

Breaking the routine is what neurobic exercising loves to do. That means "don't stay fix." Don't translate to "keep changing" in a sense when you get bored of one thing; you want to switch to the others. Try out different things to enrich the knowledge and memory span. That said, picking a new hobby stimulates all the.

Try fishing for example. The sport introduces a novelty to the mind where you need to think about how to catch a fish, the feel of water, pay attention to the weather condition, or the meal you will cook with the hooked fish.

Mastering a gadget is a smart choice in this technology era. Learn how to drive a drone, use a Go-Pro camera, subdue a video game or discover hidden features of a smart device.

15. Primitive camping

Nothing is more unexpected than an impromptu excursion. Your mission is to build a camp, collect wood sticks, start a campfire, navigate a trail and make food with the least support from modern conveniences. Feed your brain with this challenge instead of a weekend by the pool.

16. Crafting word pictures

Visualize a word in your head, make it the center. Keep on thinking about other vocabularies that begin (or end) with the same two letters. Particularly, you think of "table," it ends with "l" and "e," search your mind for words that start or end with those letters. Like "maple," "apple," "bicycle," and so on.

17. Baby crawling

When a baby crawls, they do motions like left knee up while the right arm goes up, then right knee up and left arm up. That crossing pattern gets drawn in the memory and develops different regions of the brain on both the left and the right hemispheres. We adults can take that concept to work on our brain.

By mimicking the movements, we trigger the corpus callosum connects the two halves of the brain responsible for brain maturity. You can also do full body movements where you rotate back and forth like in a transverse plane.

18. Puzzle games

Games that require efforts to connect things are extremely healthy for mental memory. Crossword, Scrabble, Jigsaw, and Sudoku are all classic puzzle games for many people to play. Preserving your brain with such kid games is not only easy to practice, but also is nothing too complicated on your regular basis.

19. Learn a new language

Speaking one or two foreign languages is one way to activate portions that lie dormant in your brain. Since learning the native tongue has disabled these parts due to its routine properties, a new linguistic will wake them up.

20. Record life

Cherish the beauty and bring what strikes your fancy into some footage. You can film anything that inspires your inner creative person and direct it into a viral video clip.

Click to follow link to get free bonus:

https://rebrand.ly/memory-cure-book

CHAPTER IV: TAKE CARE OF YOURSELF

Memory loss, as a whole, interferes in our life from odds and sods to extreme irritation. Because it involves brain work, it is something our science still keep looking to understand.

Dementia and Alzheimer's have no cure; that's is a curse. But we have a way to block its coming by putting some modifications upon our life. The best prevention is to live healthily in the young days, keep up with wholesome habits and exercise the brain to maintain its efficiency.

I hope the e-book has given you the right information to deal with the brain defection. After all, we all wish for living a full life with no suffering and being a burden when we become old.

Most importantly, treat yourself right from now on. Don't lock the stable door after the horse has bolted. And remember, if there is anyone you know catching symptoms of dementia, please give them the best support you can.

WORDS TO KNOW

Memory loss

A general term for having trouble with memorizing, not remembering past events, and being forgetful. The symptoms appear to be a part of the aging process, but can lead to forms of memory impairment.

Dementia

An "umbrella" term for a chronic disorder of the mental system resulting from a brain disease or head trauma. Memory loss is one sign of dementia.

Alzheimer's

A disease caused by the death of a series of nerve cells. It changes everything from everyday living to memory ability. It leaves defects on the neural system that will impair all daily function and cripple the patient's brain at the end.

Neurobic exercising

A workout series for the brain in which the central concept focuses on breaking the routine and giving challenges for the brain to keep improving.

Brain Scan

A test performed by a cerebral scanning machine giving out the image to show the health condition of a brain.

Mild cognitive impairment

Abbreviated to MCI. A medical condition causes memory problems, not necessarily on old people. The signs of MCI are of medium consideration since they don't affect severely on daily life.

ABOUT THE AUTHOR

Dr. Austin Coffey, MD, PhD is a physician, a nutritionist and an author. He finished his medical education at the University of Michigan. He holds master's degrees in neurosciences at the University of Miami. Finally, he has obtained a PhD doctorate in psychological and brain sciences at Johns Hopkins University. He is a fellow with the American Brain Foundation, American Academy of Neurology and the American Academy of Family Physicians. He also has a culinary degree and completed training in nutritional medicine, giving him the knowledge of nutrition as a powerful tool for disease.

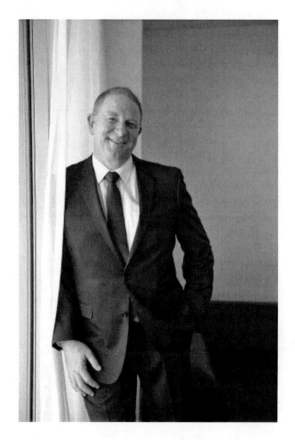

Dr. Austin Coffey

Dr. Coffey has helped thousands of patients prevent memory loss, improve their memory and regain good health. His mission is to promote the well-being of people living with memory loss and their families. He frequently leads memory loss seminars at home and abroad, which address health and nutrition issues as a guest on news broadcasts and national talk shows.

Made in United States
North Haven, CT
02 January 2022

13919688R00055